This book is dedicated to all those with Cancer

I just found out I got
Cancer

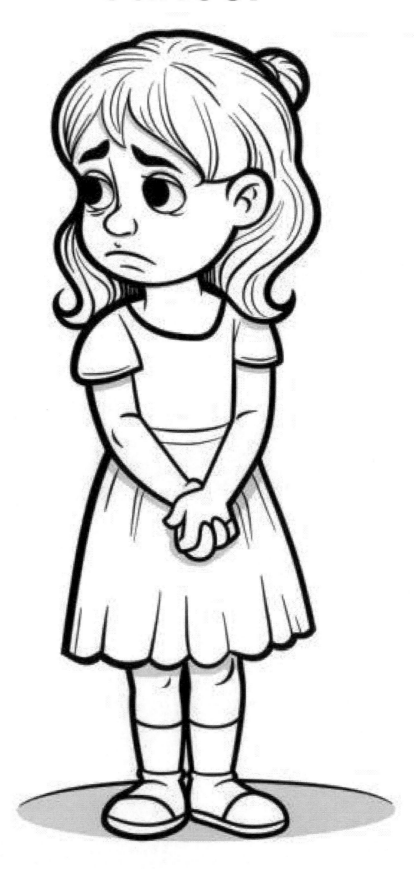

My name is Jeanie but I don't live in a bottle

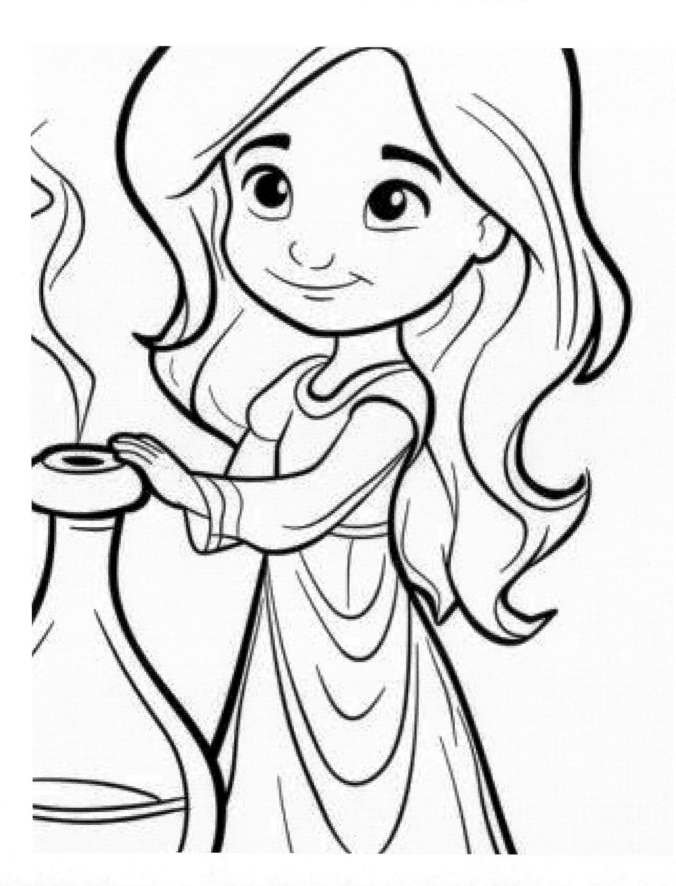

I live in the City

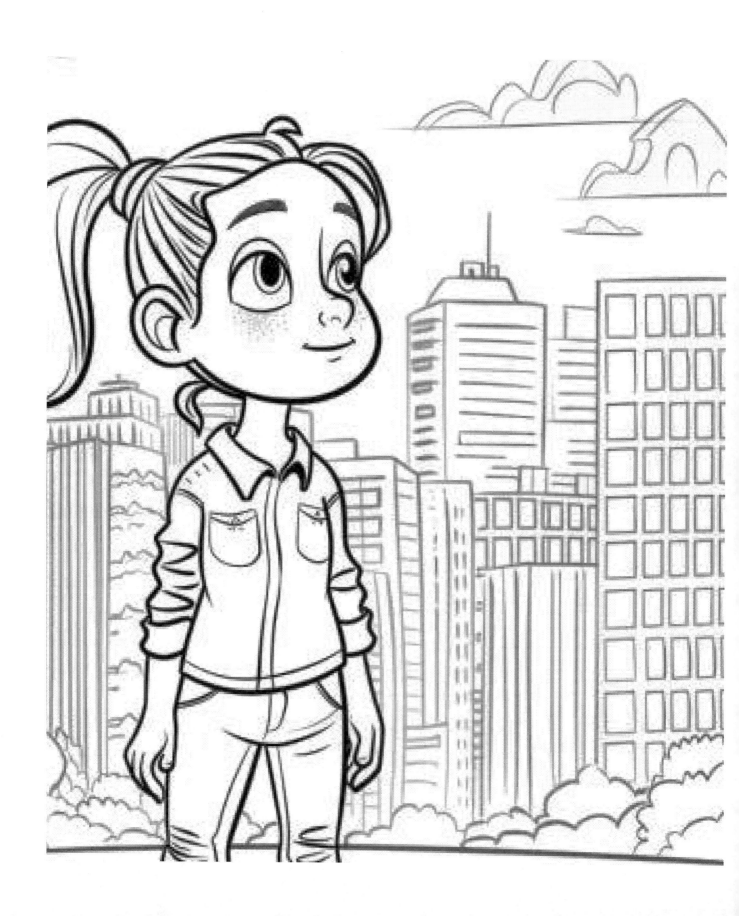

the City has lots of Buildings

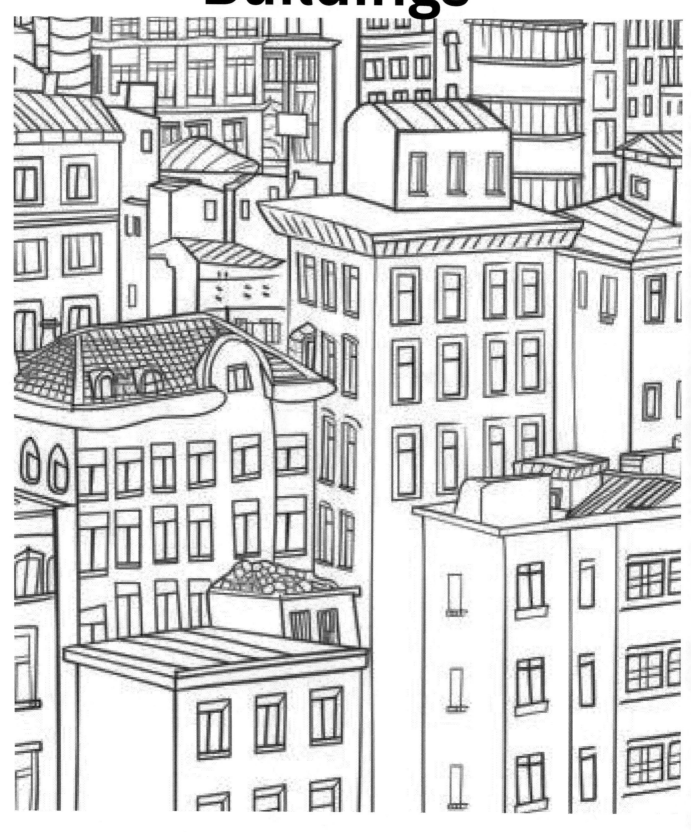

There are a lot of cars in the City

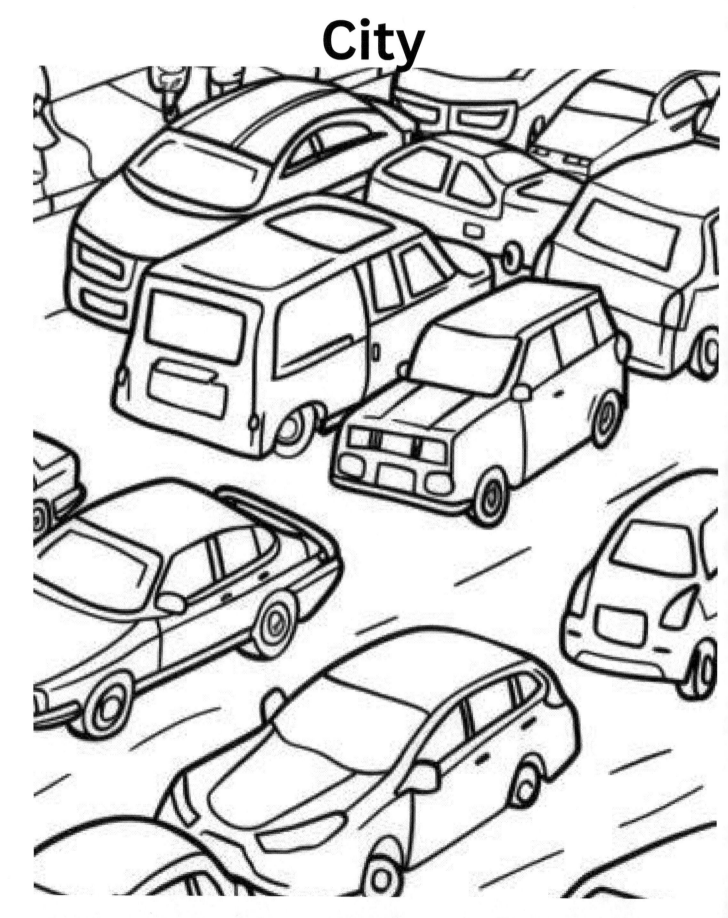

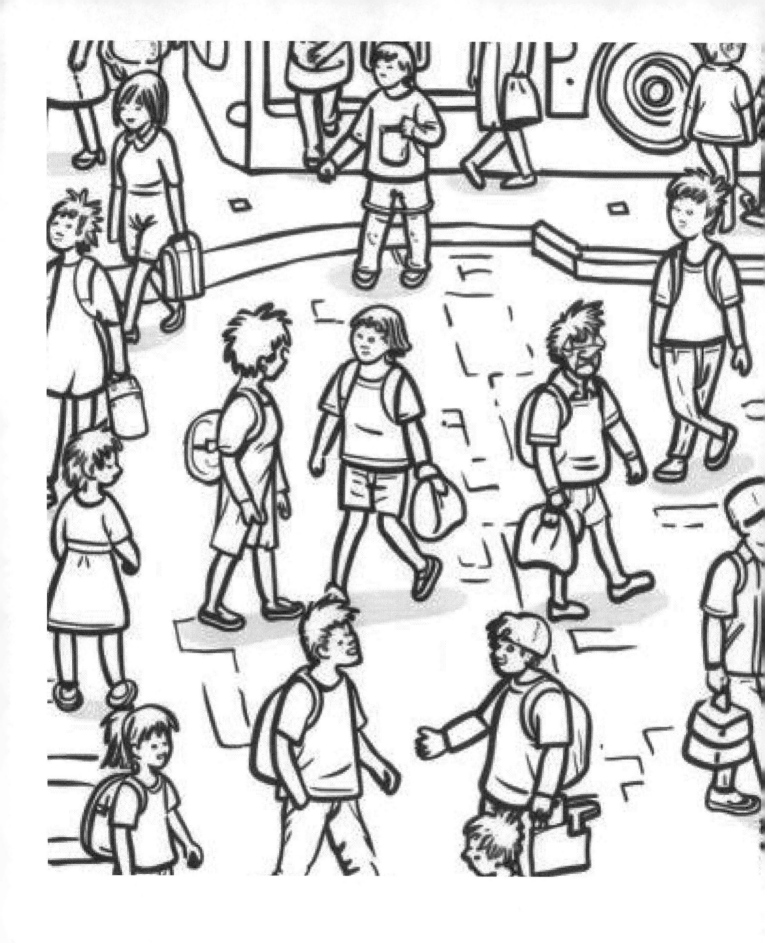

Also a lot of people

The Doctor said I have Cancer

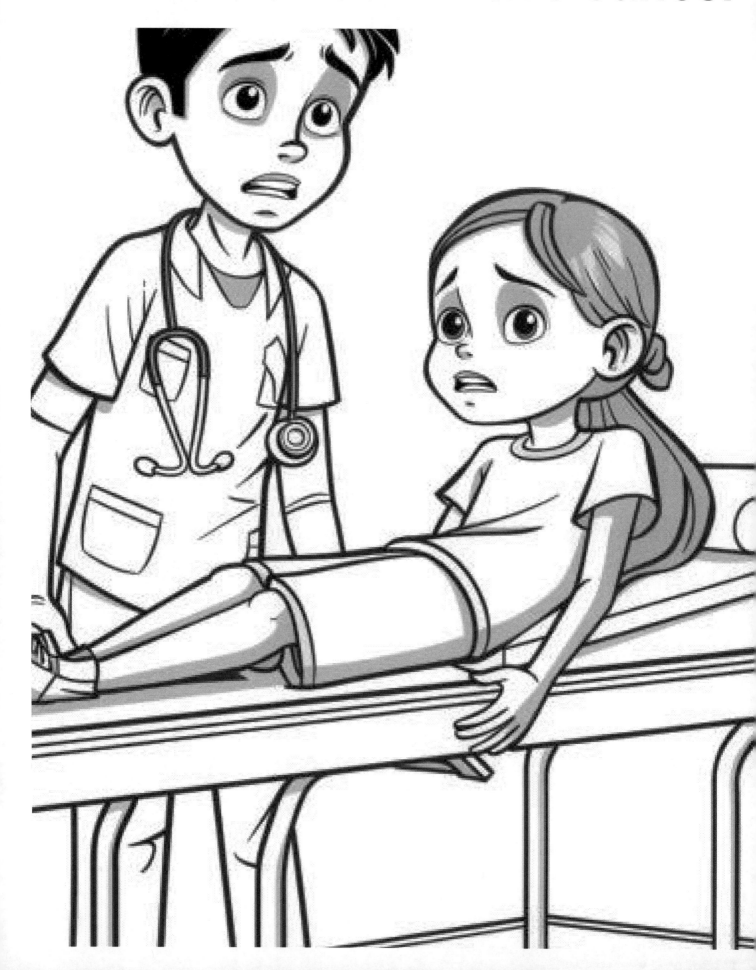

My Mom and Dad was Sad

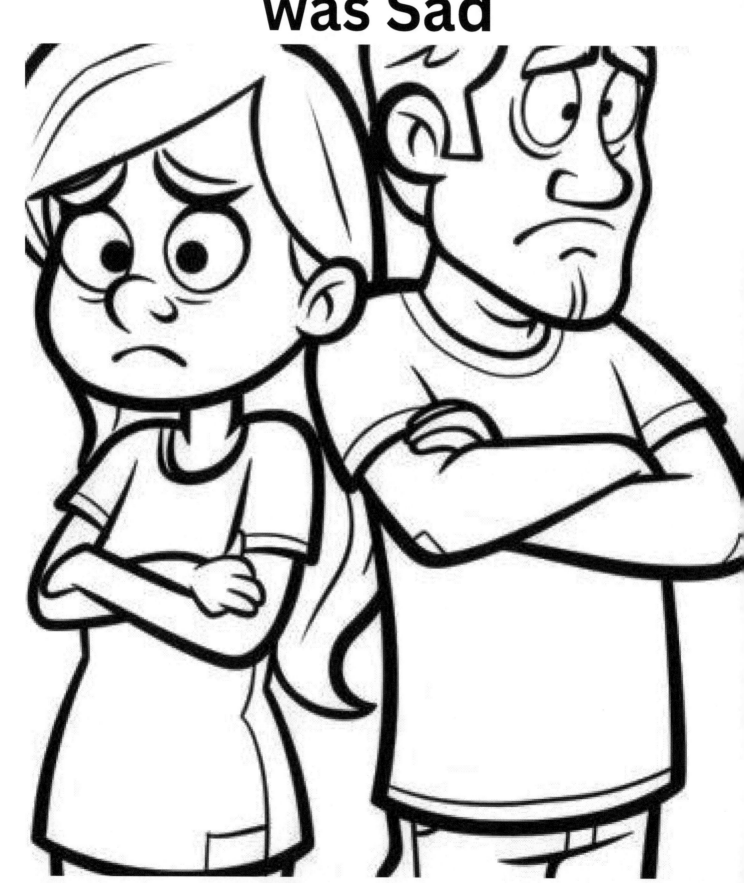

The Doctor said people die from Cancer

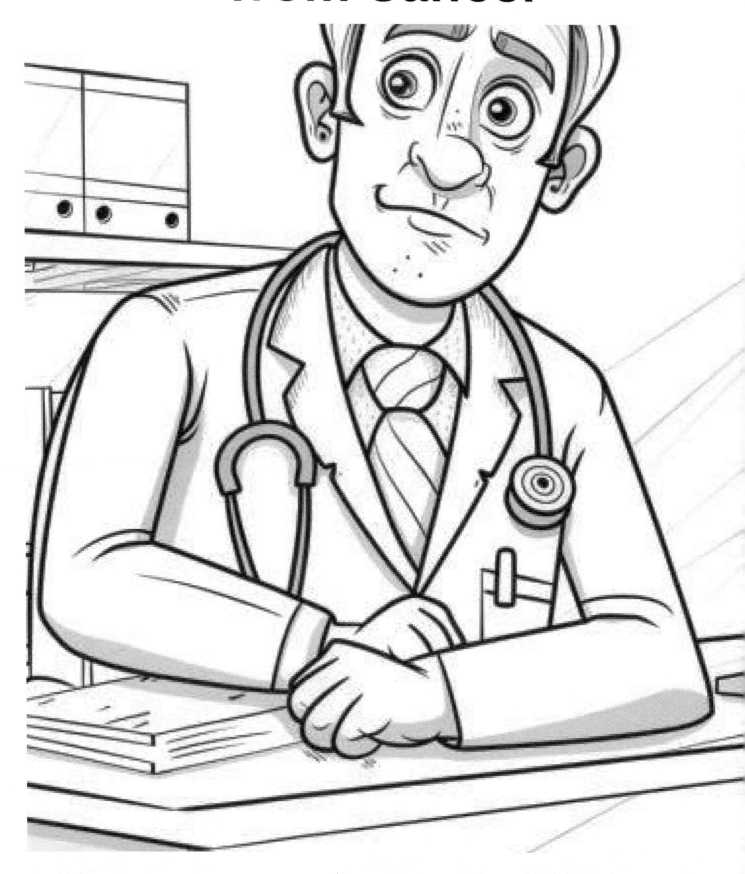

but he said I probably won't if I take the Treatments

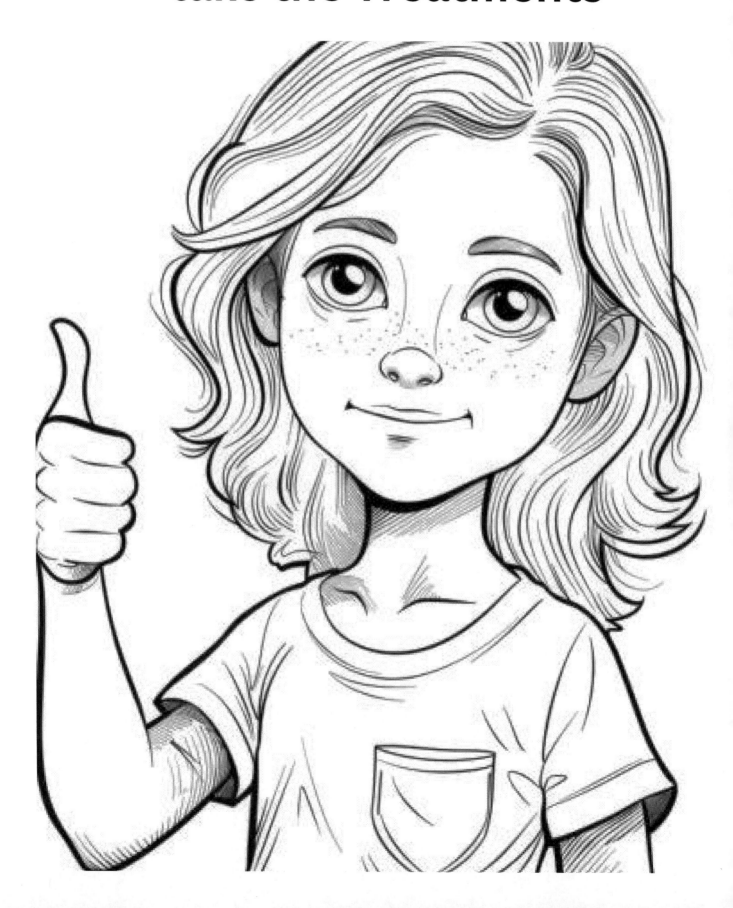

But only if God needs me

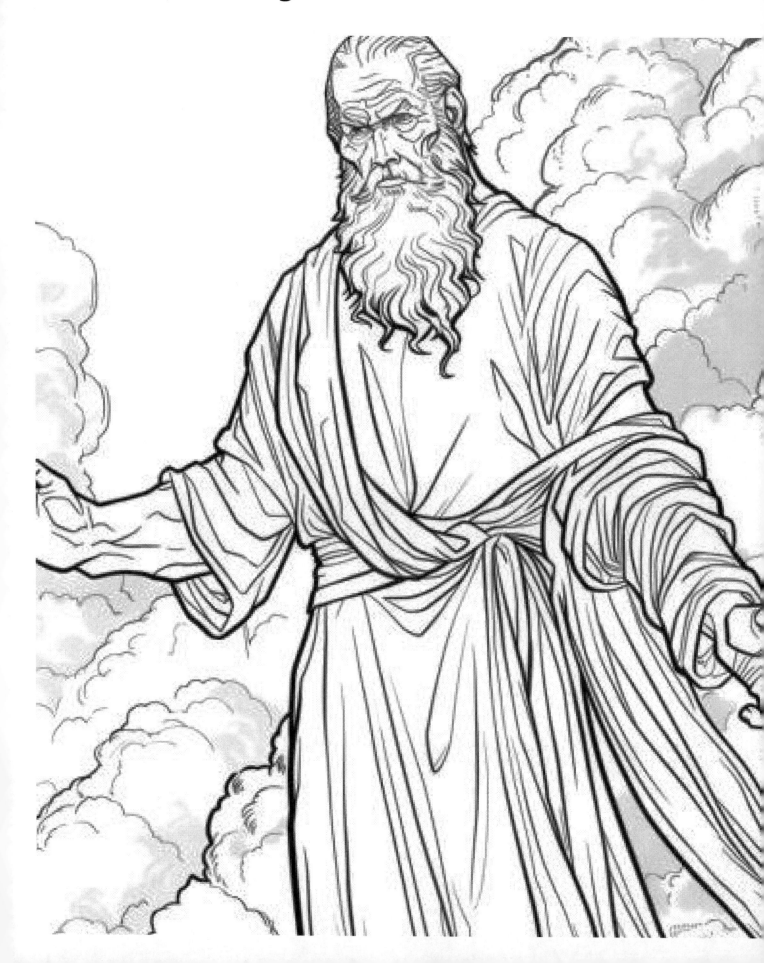

They tested my blood

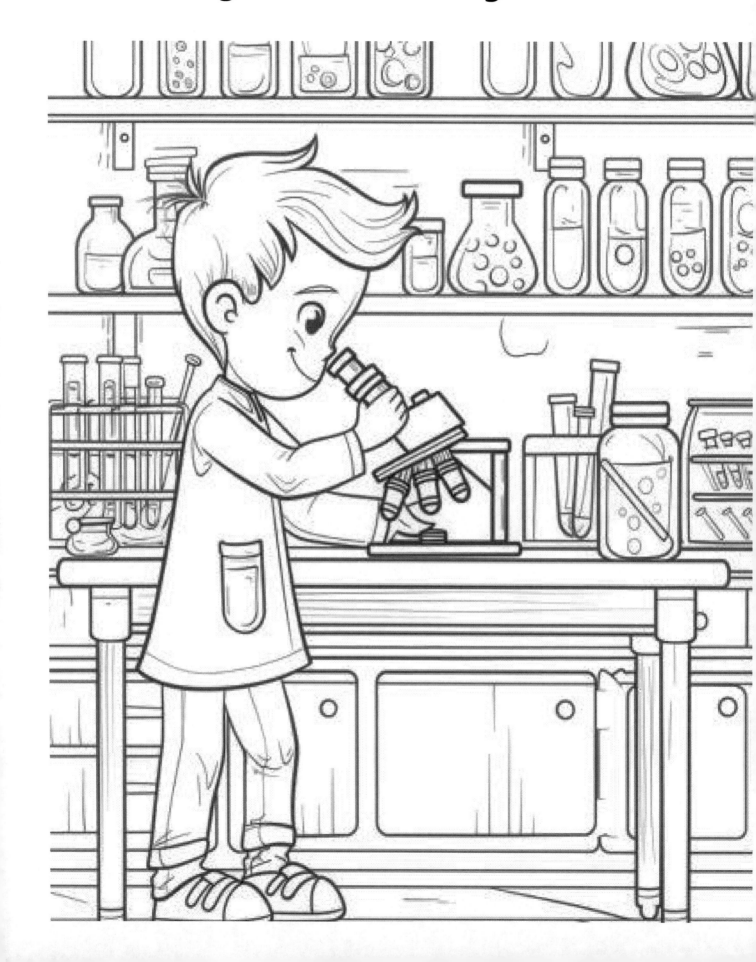

They did some other tests too

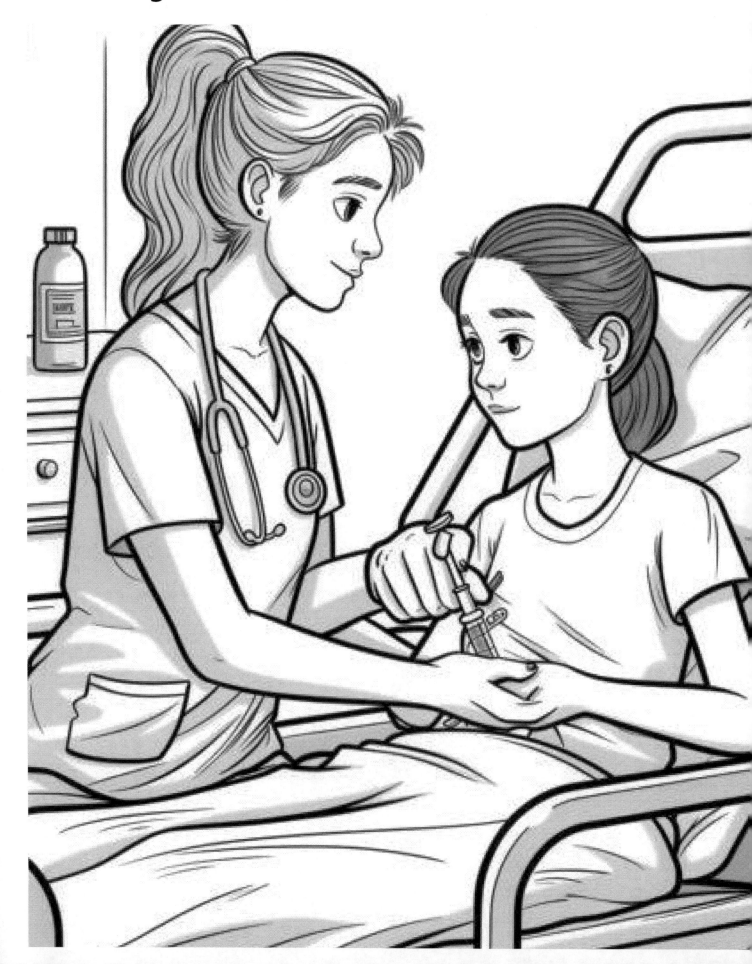

Then they said I got Cancer

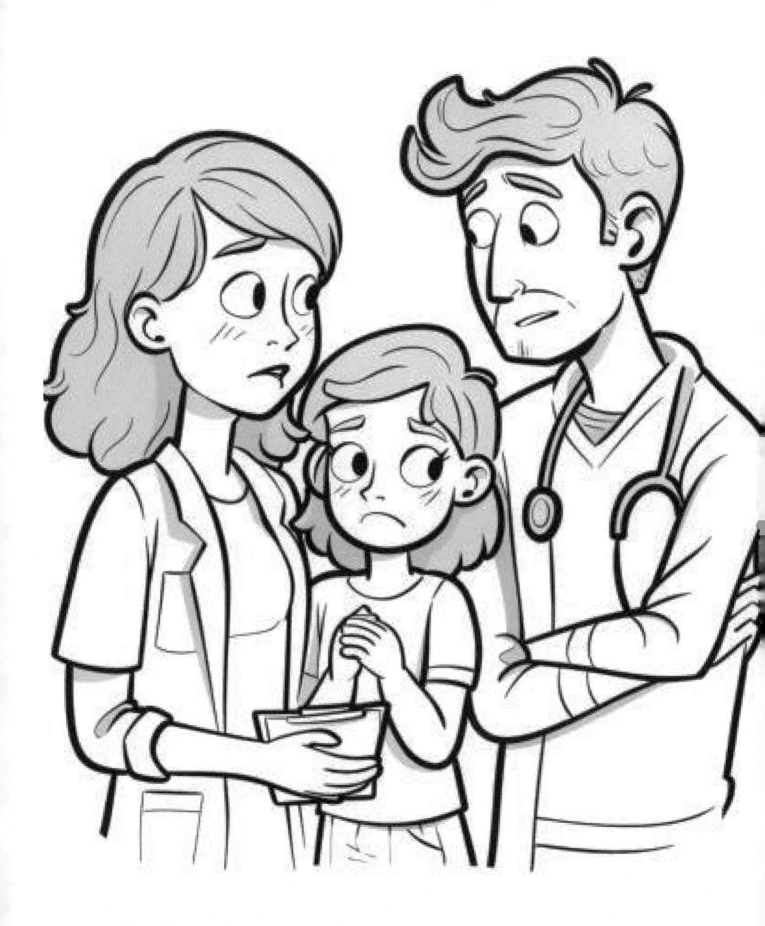

I have to take medicine through my veins

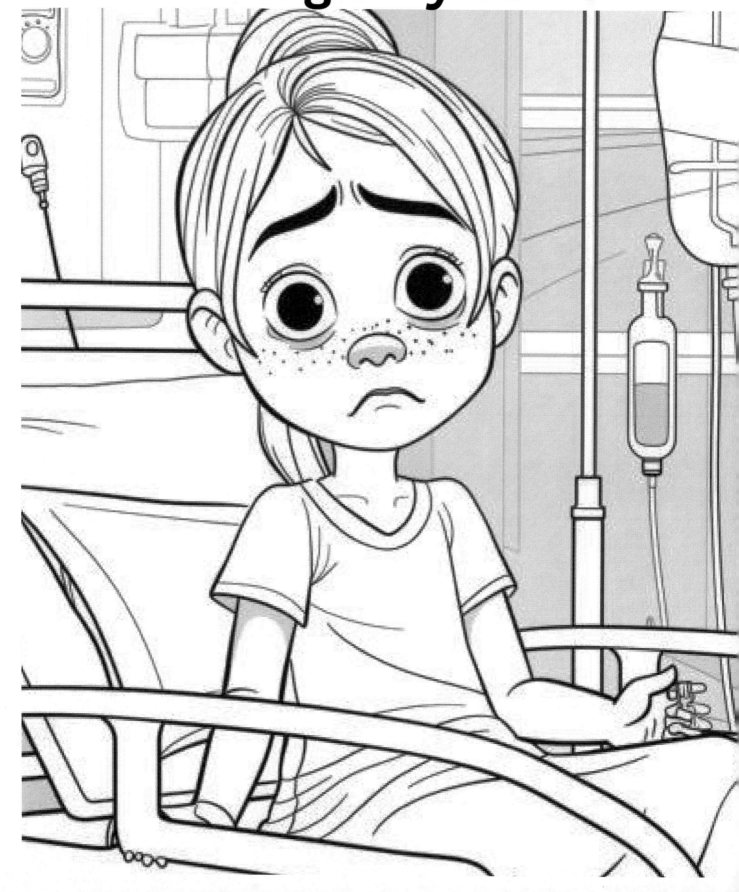

It's going to make me sick

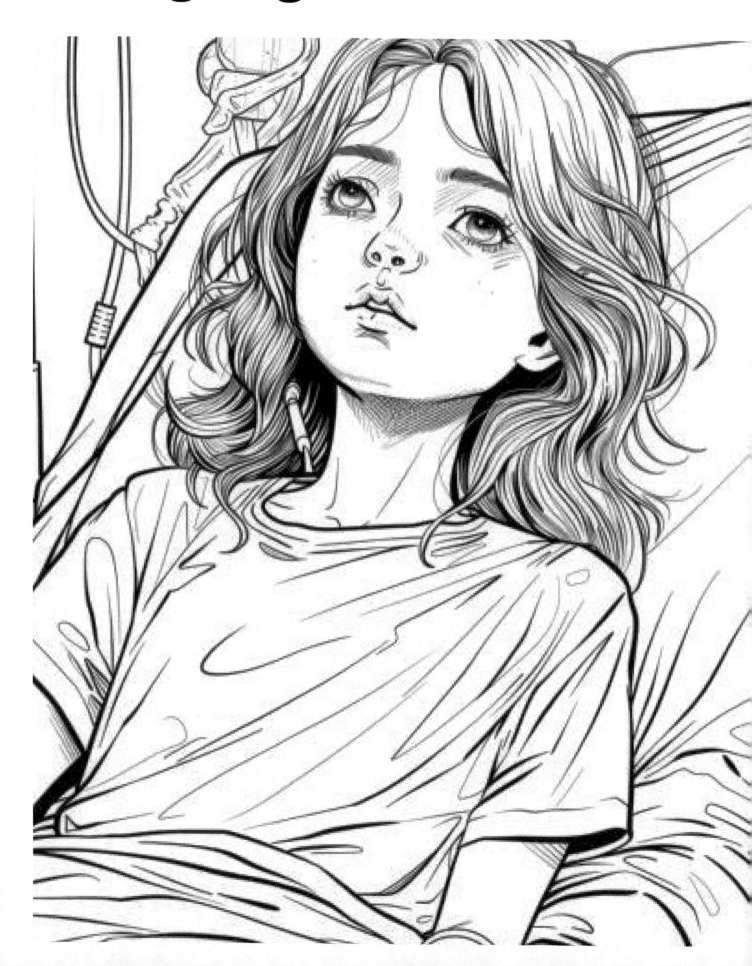

I will lose my hair

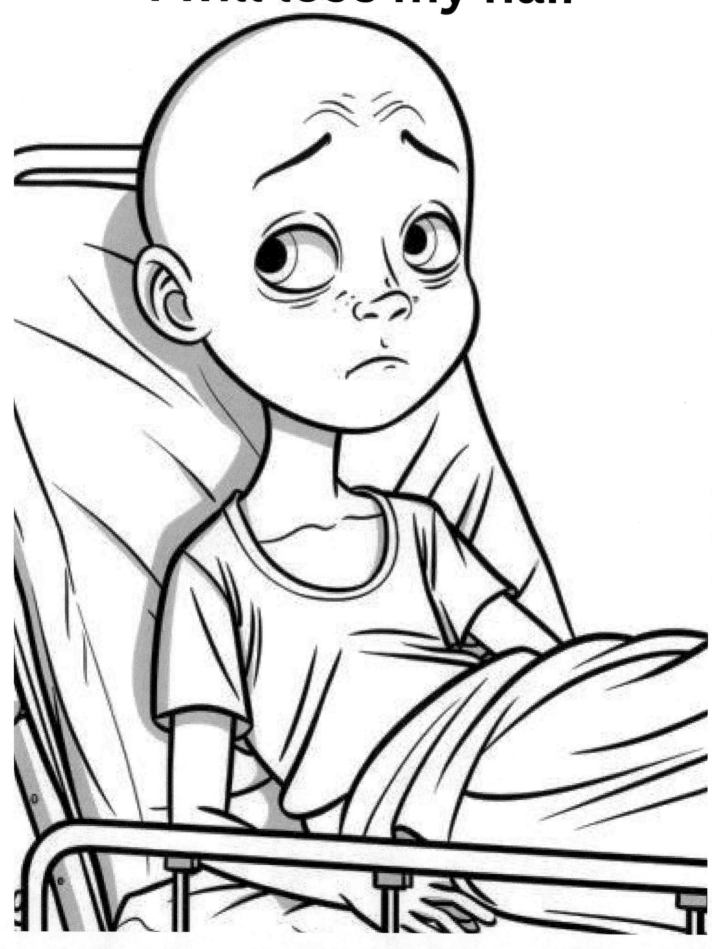

I will have to wear a hat

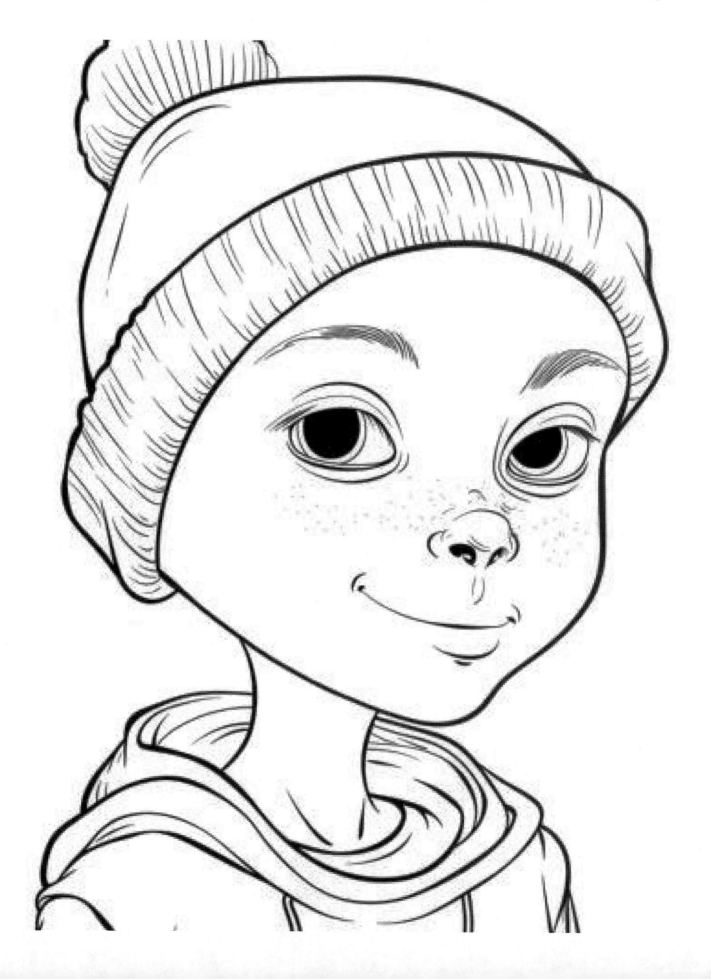

Maybe I'll get a big hat

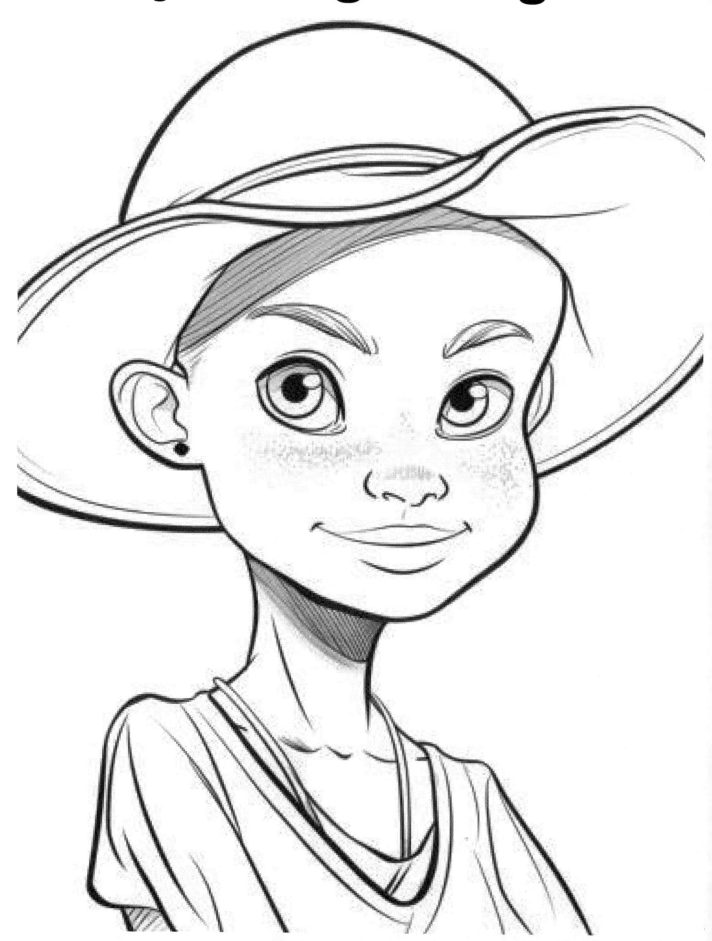

Maybe I'll get one with flowers

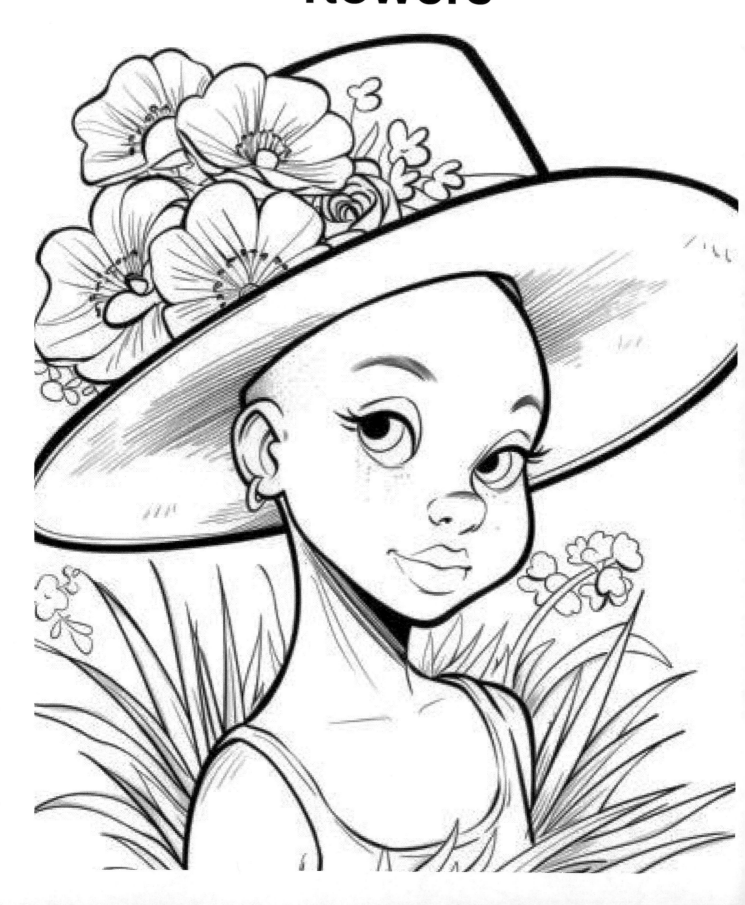

Maybe I'll get one like the Queen

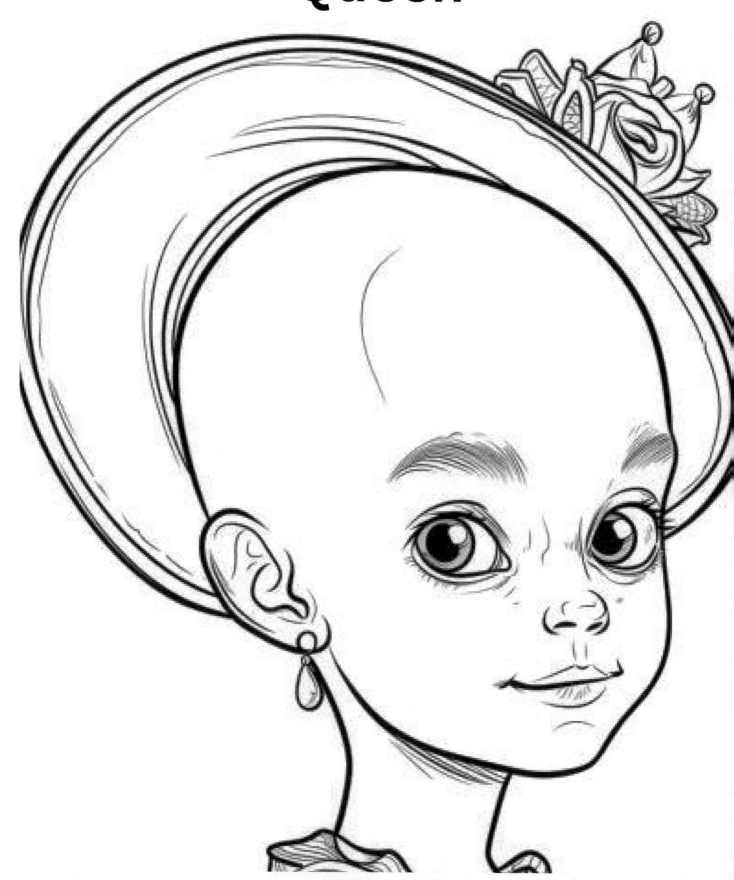

I think I'll stick to the Beanie

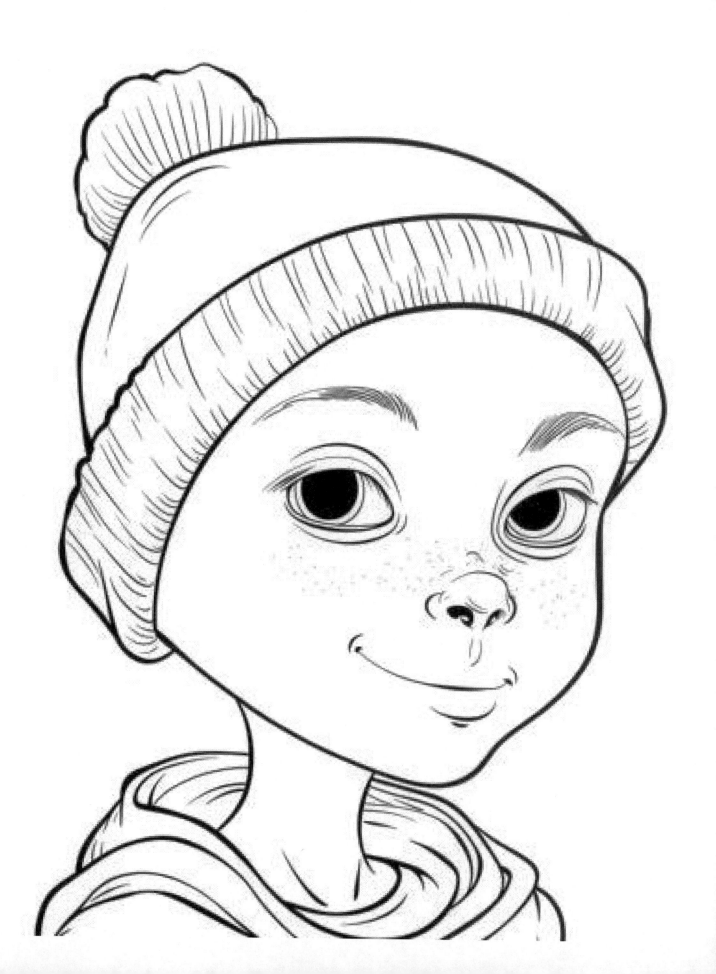

Maybe I'll wear a wig

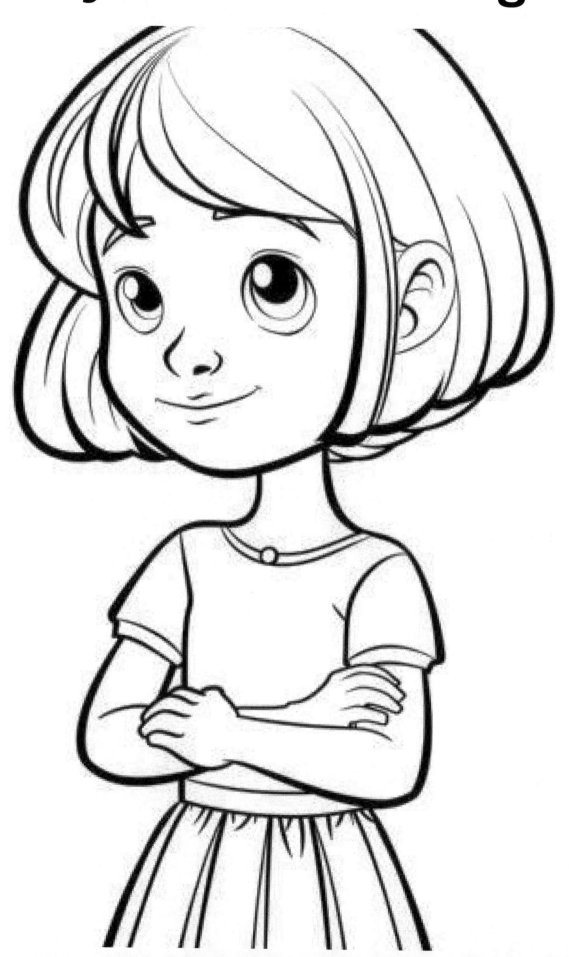

Maybe I'll get one with long flowing curls

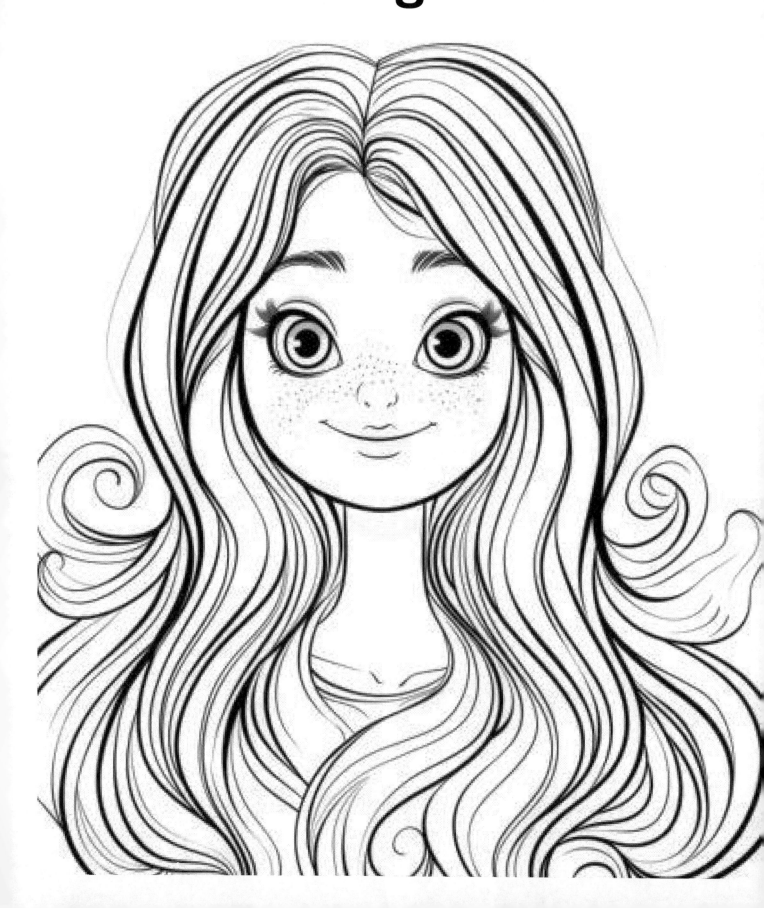

Maybe short curls

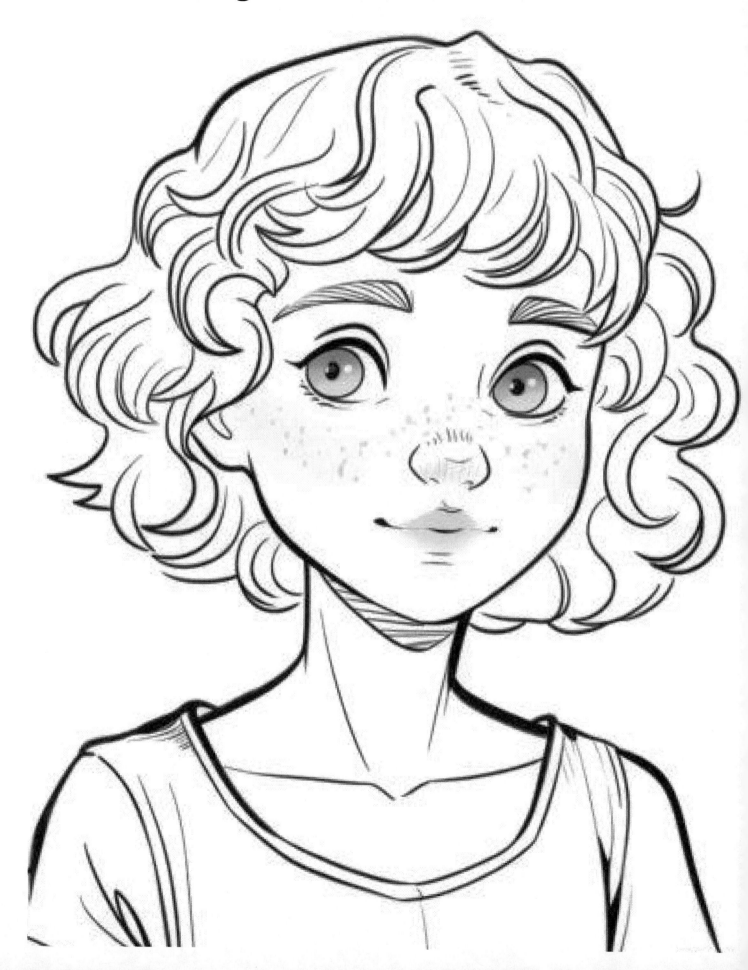

Maybe an afro

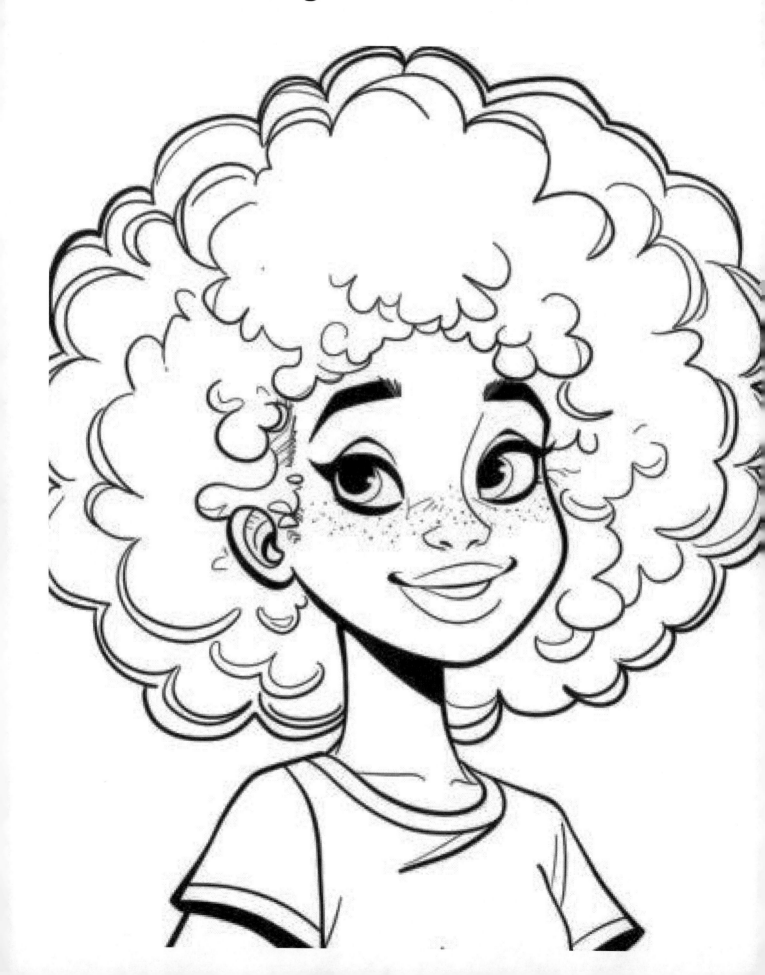

I might wear the pixie style

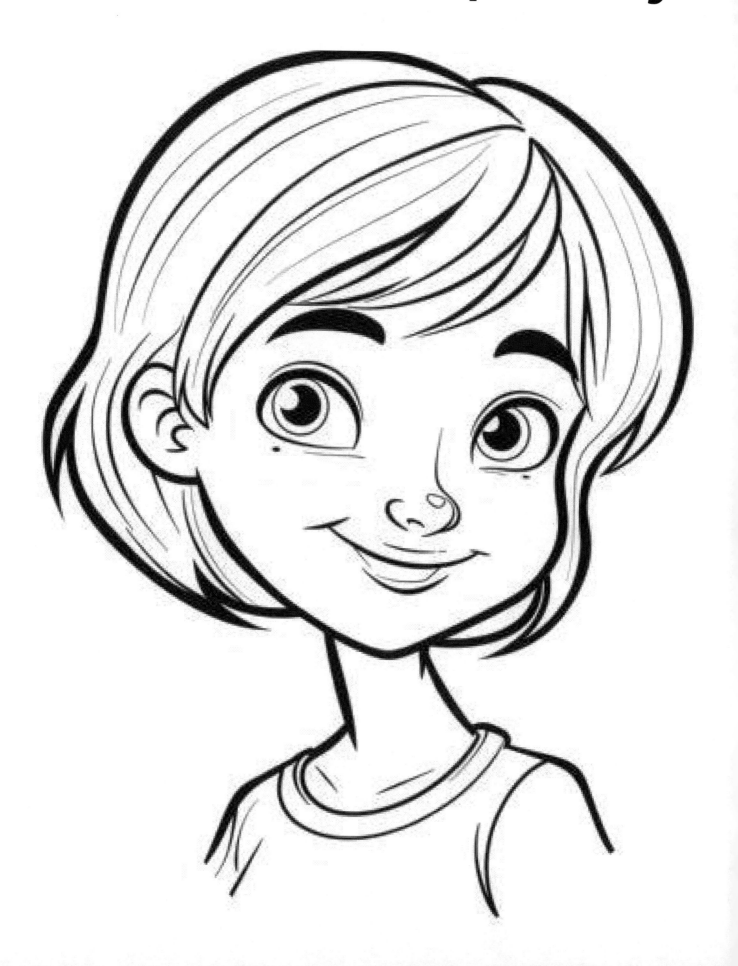

I might wear a straight shoulder length wig

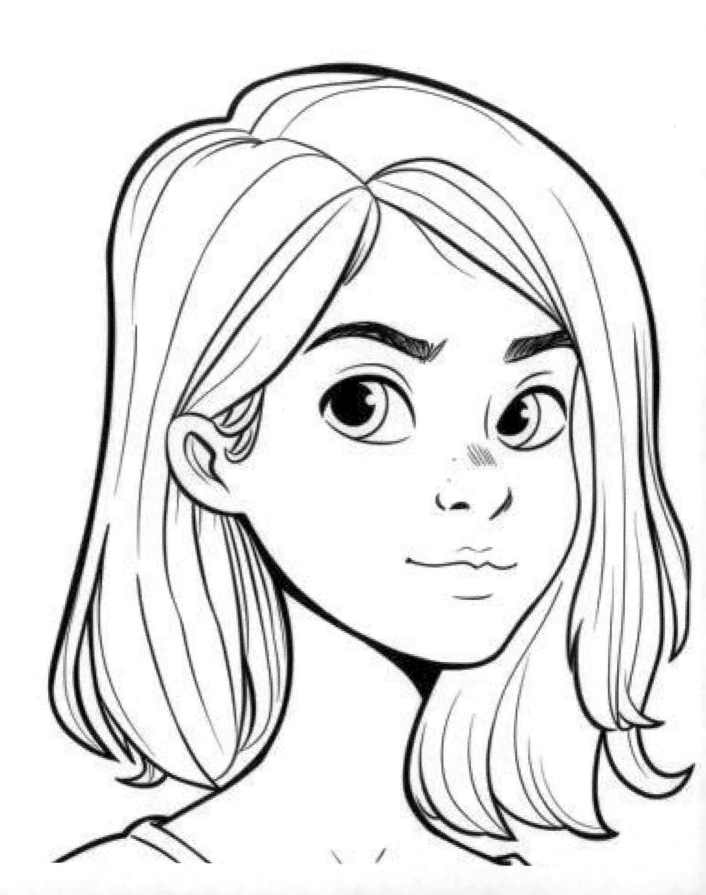

Maybe I won't wear anything

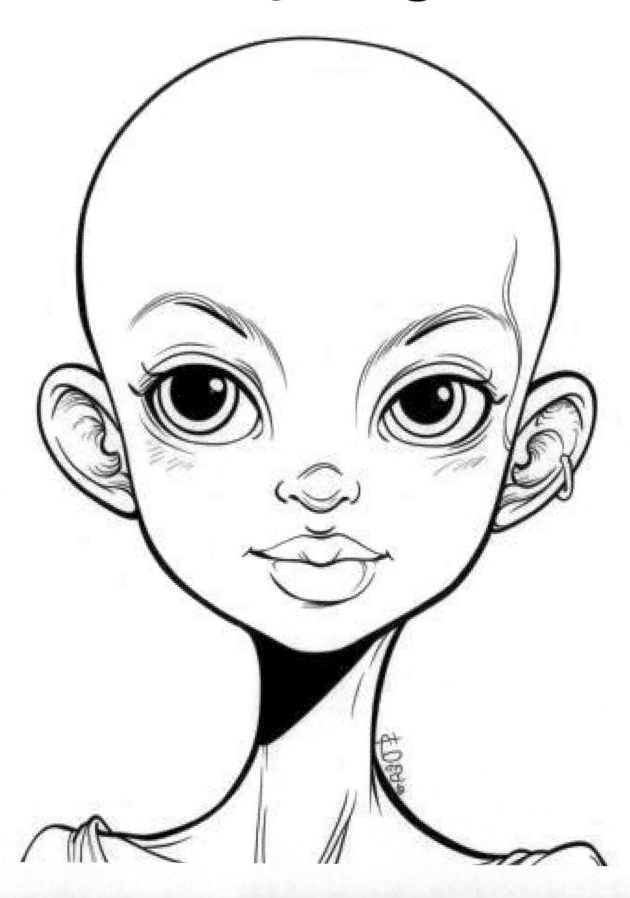

They say I won't have an appetite

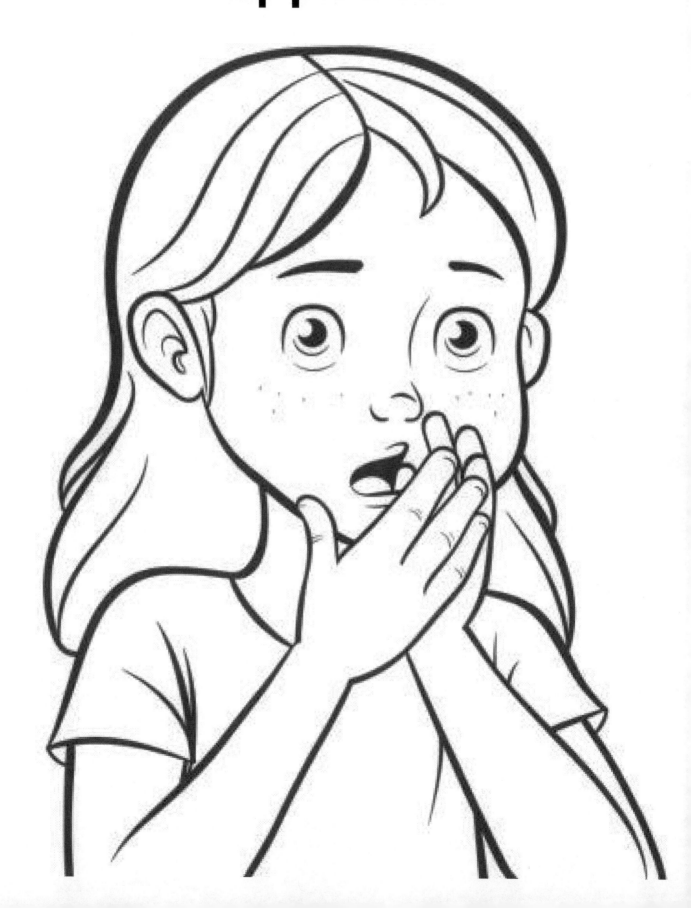

Maybe I'll just eat soup

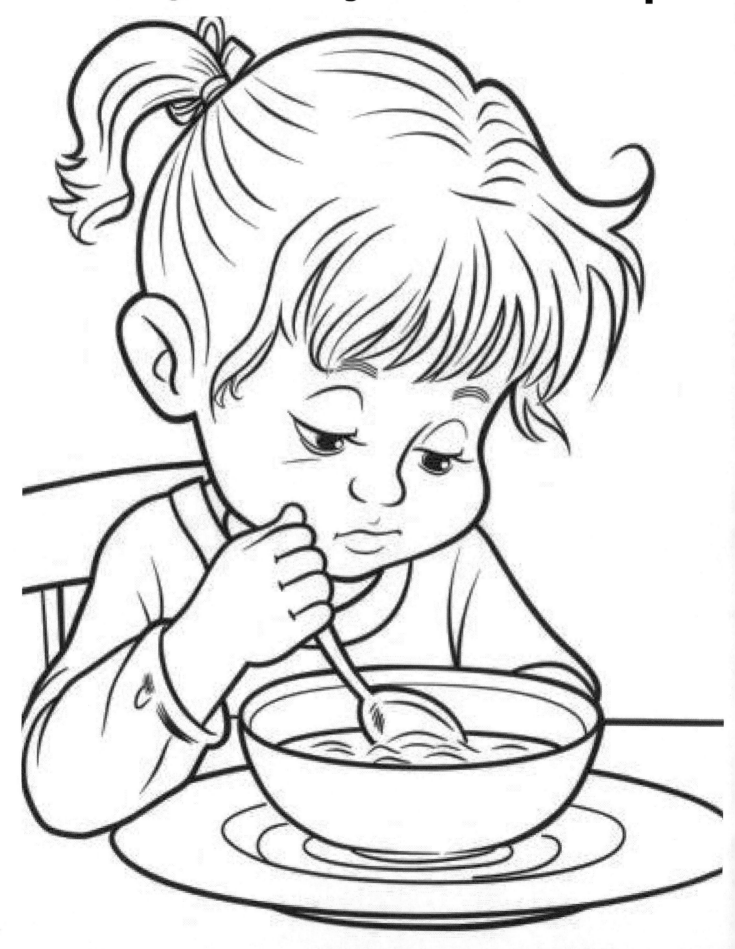

Maybe I'll eat salads

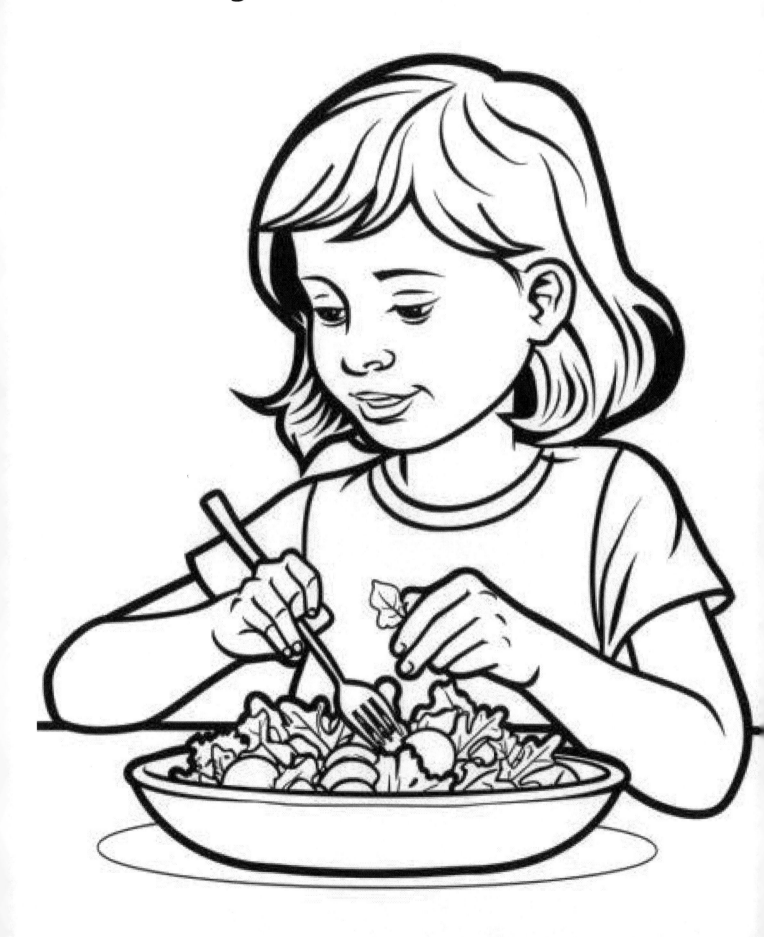

I hope I can eat a steak

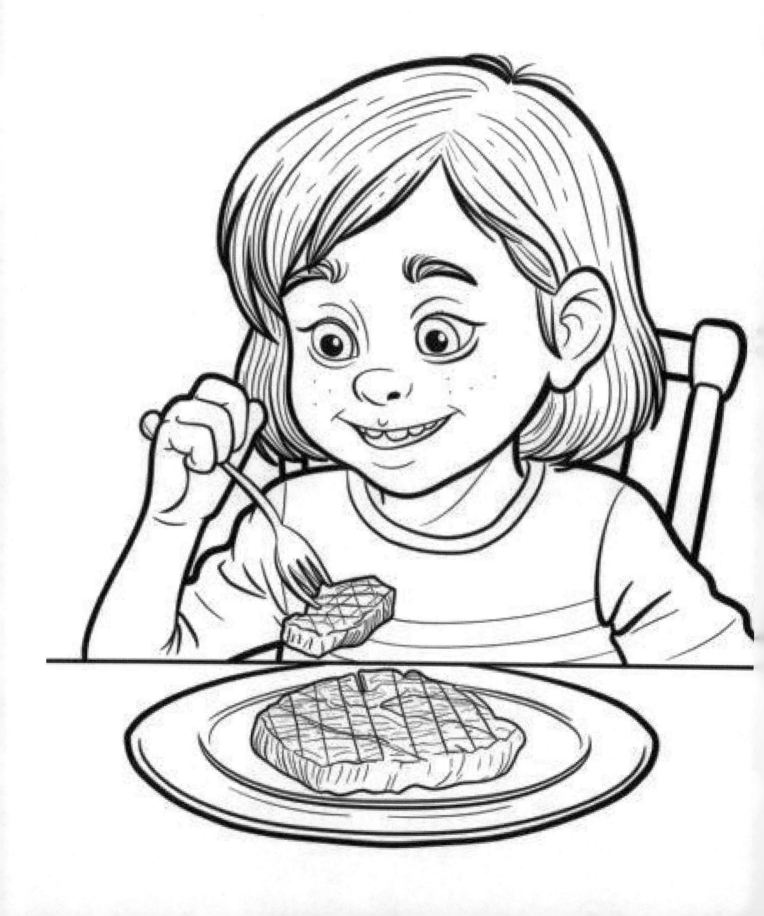

Maybe a burger and fries

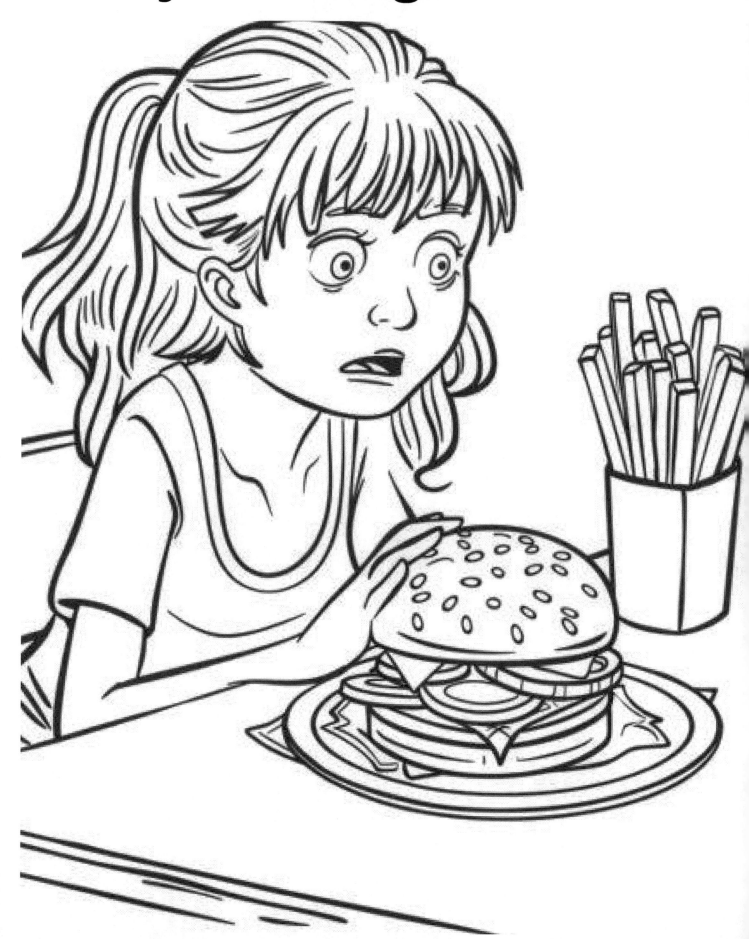

I love noodles

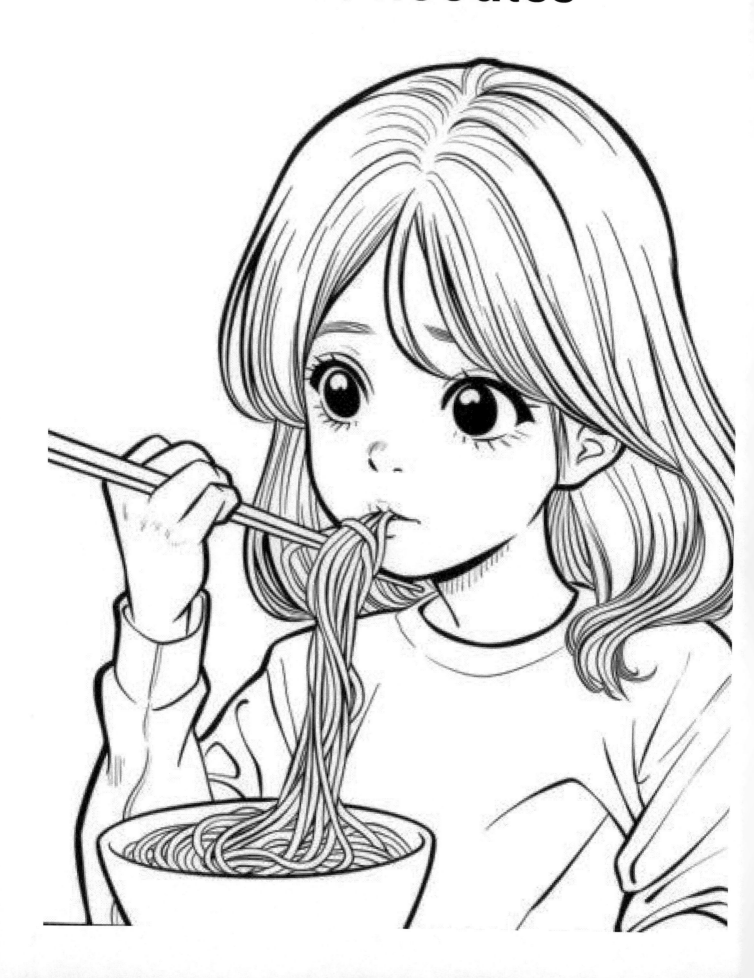

Maybe I'll just have a shake

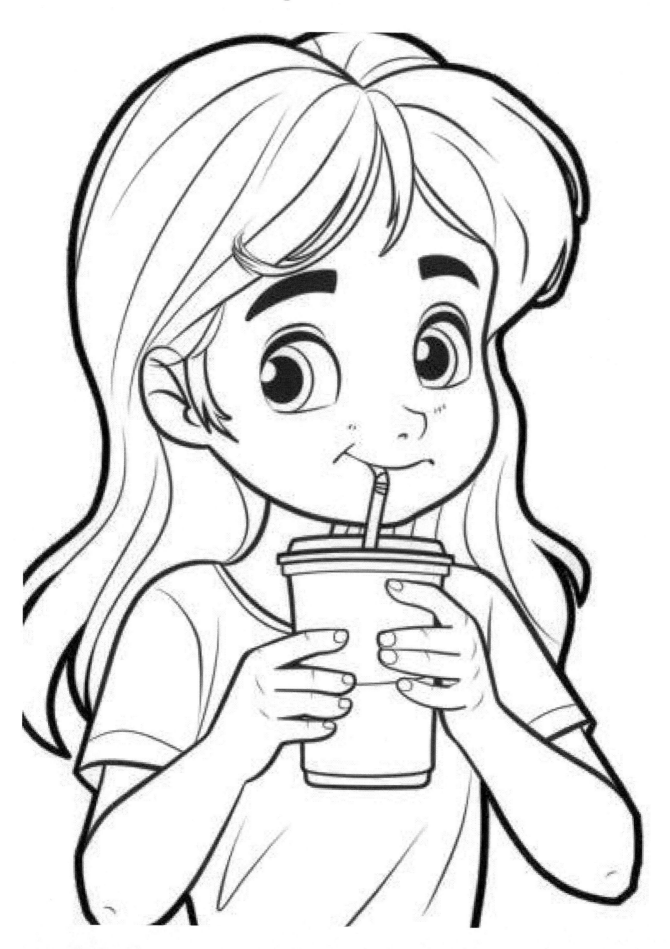

I might not be able to eat anything

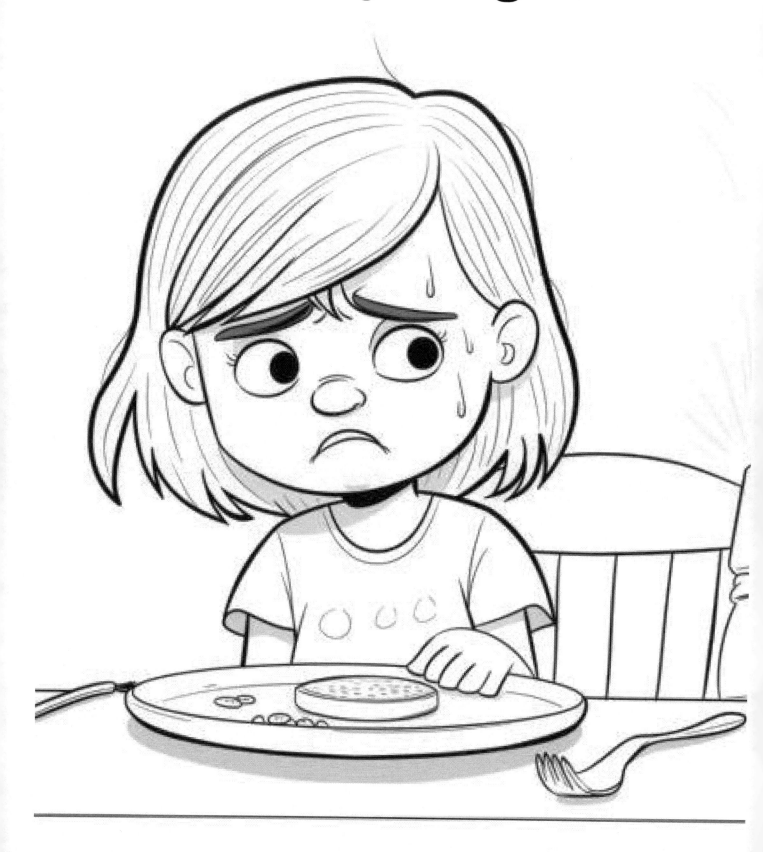

I hope I get over this soon

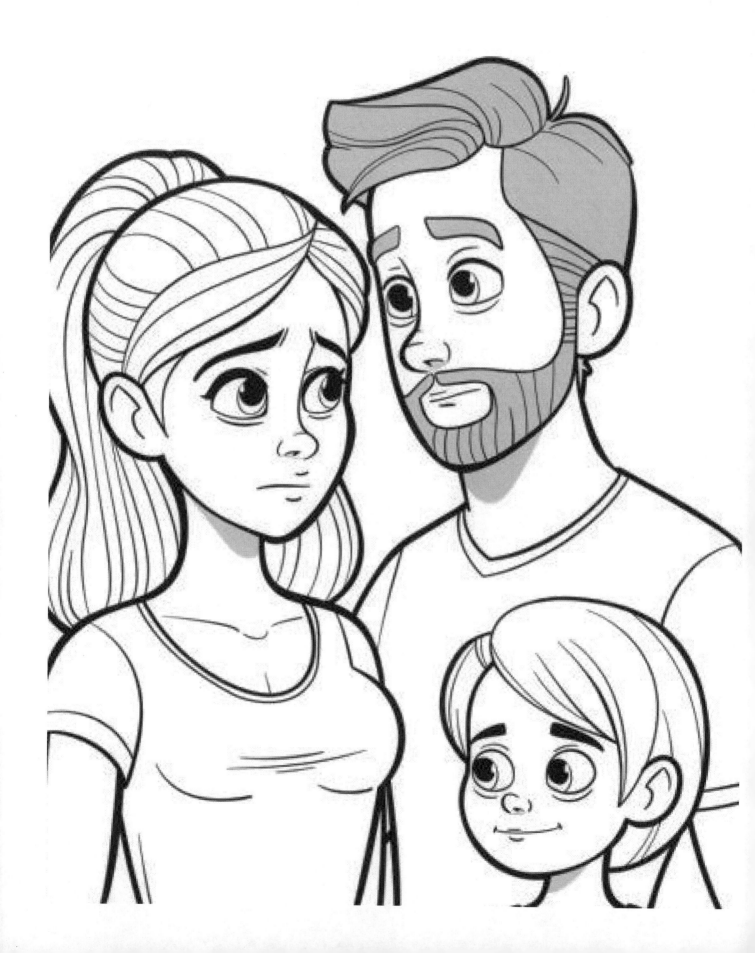

pray with my family every night

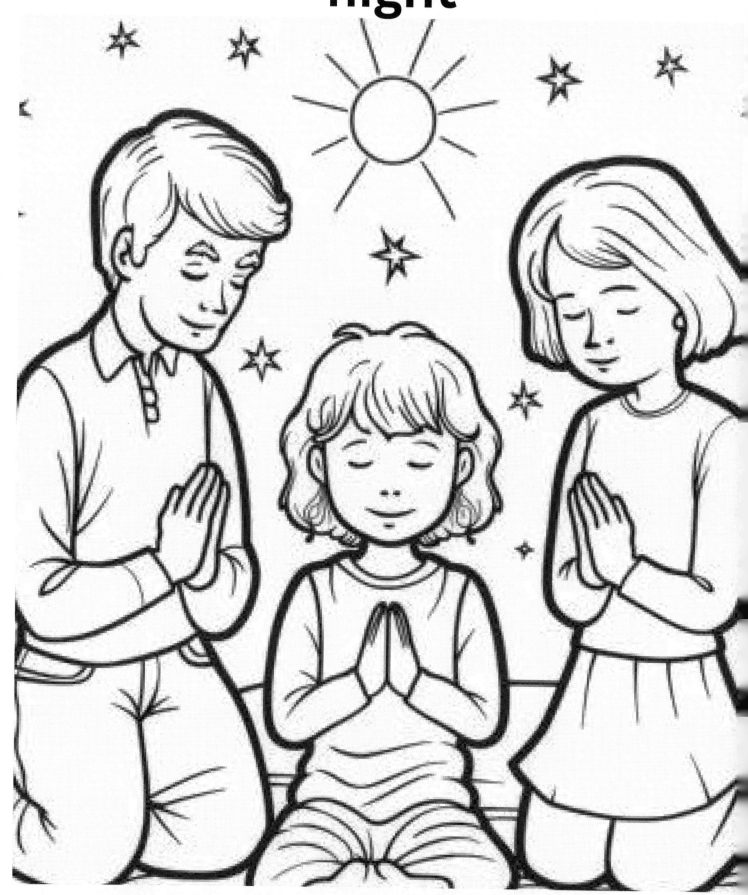

I'm a little scared but I know my parents love me

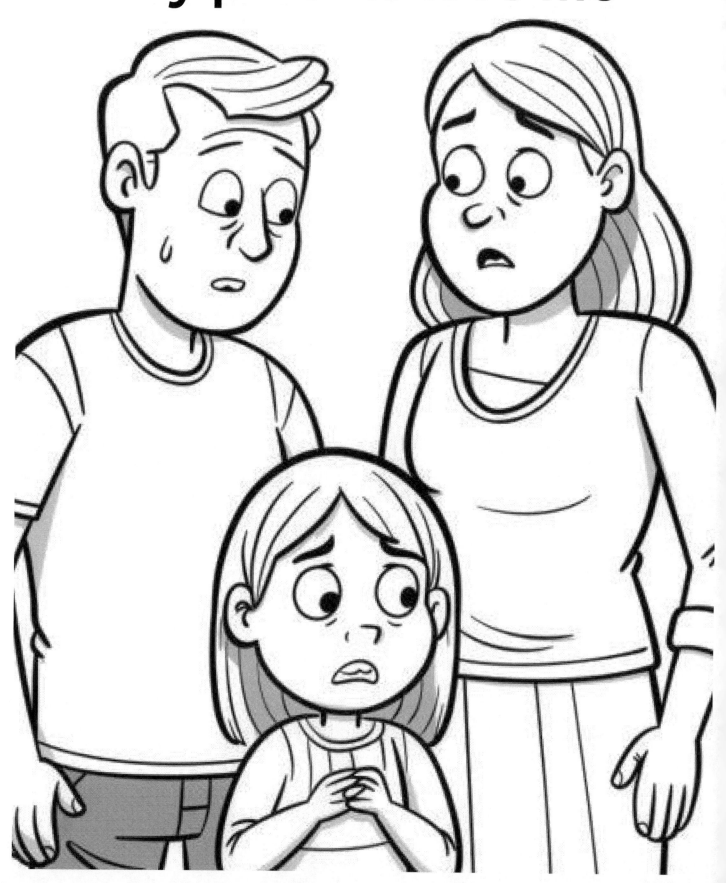

know Jesus loves me too

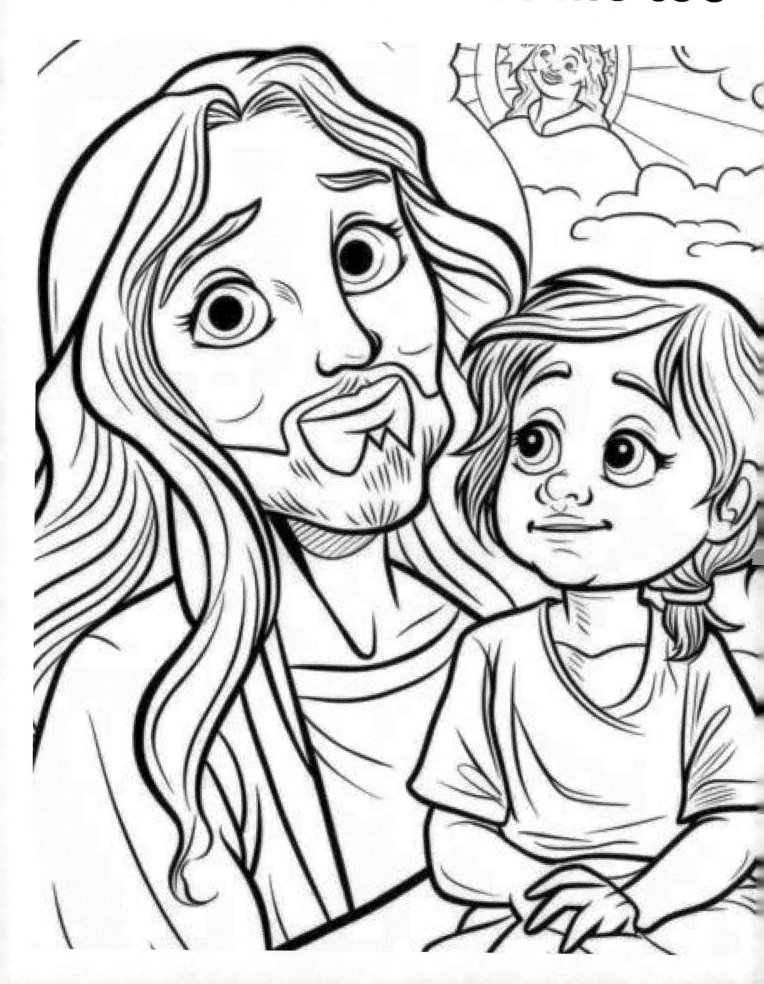

Made in the USA
Columbia, SC
17 August 2024

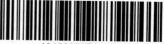

40160258R00046